ESSENTIAL GUIDE TO DYSHIDROTIC ECZEMA

Comprehensive Insights and Practical Solutions for Managing and Treating Dyshidrotic Eczema

DR. CASEY LOREN

DISCLAIMER

This book's content is only meant to be used for general informative purposes. Although the author has taken great care to ensure the content is accurate and thorough, no warranties or assurances on the information's accuracy, correctness, or reliability are provided. It is recommended that readers employ their own judgment and discretion when applying any material found in this book to their particular situation.

The information in this book is not intended to replace professional advice, nor is the author an expert in any of the subjects covered. It is recommended that readers consult with experienced professionals regarding any particular issues or concerns.

Any name that may be mentioned or referred in this book does not imply endorsement, recommendation, or relationship on the part of the author with any person, entity, good, website, or association. These references are made only for informational purposes and are not meant to be taken as recommendations or endorsements.

The information contained in this book may cause readers to suffer loss or damage, for which the author disclaims all obligation and accountability. The only people accountable for the decisions and actions taken by readers using the information presented are themselves.

Any names, characters, companies, locations, activities, occasions, and incidents referenced in this book are either made up or the result of the author's imagination. Any likeness to real people, living or dead, or to real things is entirely coincidental.

This book's content may change at any time, without prior notice, according to the author.

The onus is on the reader to verify whether there have been any updates or revisions.

The reader accepts the conditions of this disclaimer by reading this book. Please do not read this book or use its contents if you do not agree to these terms.

Table of Contents

CHAPTER 1
KNOWLEDGE ABOUT DYSHIDROTIC ECZEMA

Dyshidrotic Eczema Definition

A form of eczema that mostly affects the hands and feet is called dyshidrotic eczema, sometimes referred to as pompholyx or vesicular eczema. Small, frequently itchy blisters that can be uncomfortable are its defining feature. These blisters may be filled with liquid and present with skin scaling and redness.

Origins and Initiators

Although the precise origin of dyshidrotic eczema is unknown, a genetic and environmental component combination is thought to be responsible. The following are possible causes of dyshidrotic eczema:

- Stress or affective elements

- Contact with allergies, such as metals like cobalt or nickel

- Exposure to irritants such as solvents or detergents

- Sweating or skin that is too wet

- Variations in the temperature or weather

Signs and Symptoms

Although they can differ from person to person, dyshidrotic eczema symptoms frequently include:

- Tiny blisters on the hands, fingers, feet, or toes that are filled with fluid

- Itching, which can be moderate or quite intense

- Inflammation and redness surrounding the injured areas

Dry, chapped skin until the blisters go

- Pain or suffering, particularly if the blisters rupture or get infected

Methods of Diagnosis

Dermatologists usually perform a physical examination to diagnose dyshidrotic eczema. The physician might additionally

- Inquire about your past medical history, taking note of any allergies or skin issues.

- Use patch testing to find any possible irritants or allergies.

- In rare circumstances, obtain a skin biopsy to rule out other illnesses

Kinds and Subtypes

Although it usually affects the hands and feet, dyshidrotic eczema can also appear in other body areas. Dyshidrotic eczema variants include:

Limiting to the palms of the hands and soles of the feet is vesicular palmoplantar eczema.

- Dyshidrotic eczema of the fingers: A condition that only affects the fingertips and is frequently brought on by contact with allergens or irritants

- Pompholyx: Another word for the characteristic blisters associated with dyshidrotic eczema that is used interchangeably with it

Danger Elements

The following variables may make dyshidrotic eczema more likely to occur:

- A family history of allergies or eczema

- A personal history of skin conditions or various forms of eczema

- Exposure to allergens or irritants at work, such as for hair stylists or healthcare personnel

- Emotional or lifestyle stressors

Distinguishing Dyshidrotic Eczema from Other Skin Disorders

It is possible to differentiate dyshidrotic eczema from other skin disorders by looking for certain symptoms and characteristics. As an illustration:

- The absence of a more widespread rash and the presence of tiny blisters set it apart from contact dermatitis.

It differs from fungal diseases in that it does not exhibit common fungal patterns such as ringworm.

- Small, fluid-filled blisters are the hallmark of dyshidrotic eczema, in contrast to the thick, scaly patches that frequently accompany psoriasis.

Statistics and Prevalence

About 5 to 20% of instances of hand eczema are dyshidrotic eczema, making it a moderately common condition. Although it can afflict anyone of any age, persons between the ages of 20 and 40 are more likely to experience it. Additionally, women are somewhat more likely than men to get dyshidrotic eczema.

Effect on Life Quality

The quality of life can be significantly impacted by having dyshidrotic eczema. Itching and pain are some of the symptoms that might interfere with sleep, work, and everyday activities. Because the blisters are visible, some people may experience mental discomfort or social disengagement as a result of feeling self-conscious or embarrassed.

Myths and False Beliefs

Regarding dyshidrotic eczema, there are several myths and misunderstandings, including:

Myth: It may spread easily. Dyshidrotic eczema is not transmissible by physical touch.

Myth: Only inadequate hygiene is to blame. The main causes of dyshidrotic eczema are hereditary and environmental, though cleanliness can also be a factor.

Myth: There is a permanent cure. There is no known cure for dyshidrotic eczema, even though treatments can effectively manage symptoms.

It is essential to comprehend these facets of dyshidrotic eczema to provide appropriate care and assistance to those who suffer from it.

CHAPTER 2

SKIN ANATOMY

Layers of the Skin

1. **Epidermis**: The skin's outermost layer, is mainly made up of epithelial cells. It protects the skin from the elements, controls water loss, and contains the melanocytes that give skin its color.

2. **Dermis**: The dermis, which is situated beneath the epidermis, is home to hair follicles, sweat glands, blood vessels, and nerves. It is essential for wound healing and gives the skin structural support.

3. **Hypodermis**: Also referred to as the subcutaneous layer, it is made up of connective tissue and fat cells. The hypodermis serves the body's needs as an energy reserve, cushion, and insulator.

The Skin's Functions

1. **Protection**: Internal organs are shielded from infections, ultraviolet light, and mechanical trauma by the skin, which serves as a physical barrier.

2. **Sensation**: Touch, pressure, warmth, and pain are all sensed by nerve endings in the skin.

3. **Thermoregulation**: By releasing or storing heat as needed, blood vessels and sweat glands assist in controlling body temperature.

4. **Excretion**: Sweat glands control electrolyte balance and remove waste items.

The Skin Barrier: Its Significance

The epidermis forms the skin barrier, which is essential for preserving the health of the skin. To preserve homeostasis, it stops water loss, protects against allergens and pathogens, and controls immune responses.

Sweat Glands' Function

Through the production of sweat, sweat glands—including eccrine and apocrine glands—play a critical role in controlling body temperature. Apocrine glands, which are mostly located in the groin and armpits, release a thicker fluid that is impacted by stress, whereas eccrine glands, which are dispersed throughout the body, secrete perspiration to cool the skin.

Skin's Immune System

Numerous immune cells, including macrophages, T cells, and Langerhans cells, which fight infections and control inflammatory reactions, are found in the skin. Eczema and other immune response dysregulation can result in medical disorders.

Nervous System and Skin Health Associated with It

Skin nerves are responsible for controlling glandular activities, blood flow, and sensory information transmission. Stress and neurological disorders can hurt skin health, making eczema worse.

Elements Affecting Skin Condition

1. **Environmental Factors**: Temperature swings, pollution, humidity, and UV radiation can all have an impact on skin health.

2. **Lifestyle Decisions**: Skin condition is influenced by sleep patterns, nutrition, hydration, and skincare practices.

3. **Genetics**: Certain people are predisposed to certain skin disorders, such as eczema.

4. **Medical Conditions**: Chronic illnesses, autoimmune diseases, and hormone imbalances can all affect the health of your skin.

Microbiome of the Skin

A wide variety of bacteria, fungi, and other microorganisms make up the skin's microbiome. Skin health depends on a balanced microbiome since it affects barrier function and immunological responses.

Skin Moisture and pH Balance

The pH balance of the skin, which is normally slightly acidic, controls microbial development and aids in preserving the integrity of the skin barrier. Sufficient moisture content is essential for skin hydration, suppleness, irritation, and dryness prevention.

The Signs of Ageing Skin

Wrinkles, sagging, and an increased susceptibility to environmental damage can be caused by aging processes such as decreased collagen formation, decreased skin elasticity, and slower cell turnover. Good eating, lifestyle, and skincare practices can lessen these impacts.

Effective management of disorders such as dyshidrotic eczema requires a fundamental understanding of these aspects of skin architecture, function, and maintenance. Would you like further information about any particular topic?

CHAPTER 3

ECZEMA CAUSES AND PREVENTIVE MEASURES

Typical Causes of Dyshidrotic Eczema

1. **Climatic Factors**:

- Flare-ups can be brought on by exposure to harsh chemicals such as solvents, detergents, or certain metals.

- Frequent hand washing without adequate moisturization or extended exposure to water might also act as triggers.

- The risk may be higher for some jobs if they need a lot of hand washing or expose workers to irritants.

2. **Nutritional Stressors**:

Some people may have flare-ups because of certain foods, such as citrus fruits, dairy products, or gluten.

- In some circumstances, drinking alcohol or caffeine can make symptoms worse.

3. **Irritants and Allergens**:

- Dust mites, mold, pollen, and pet dander are examples of allergens that can aggravate eczema symptoms.

- Fragrances, fabric softeners, and harsh soaps are examples of irritants that can cause flare-ups.

4. **Emotional and Stress Triggers**:

- The immune system might be weakened and eczema bouts can be triggered by emotional stress, worry, or sadness.

- Stress-reduction methods such as yoga, meditation, or counseling may be beneficial.

5. The **climate conditions**:

- Dry weather, high humidity, and extreme temperatures can exacerbate eczema symptoms.

These effects can be lessened by applying moisturizers or humidifiers and covering up with proper clothing to protect the skin.

6. **Skincare and Personal Hygiene Products**:

- The skin might get irritated by using abrasive soaps, shampoos, or skincare products that contain alcohol or scents.

- Avoiding harsh, scented items and applying moisturizer frequently will help avert flare-ups.

Preventative Actions

1. **Changes to Lifestyle**:

Reducing exposure to allergens, harsh chemicals, and stressful environments can help avoid exacerbations of eczema.

- Eating a diet high in fruits, vegetables, and omega-3 fatty acids will help to maintain good skin health overall.

2. **Establishing a Setting Free from Triggers**:

- Dryness and irritation can be avoided by following good hand hygiene procedures and not washing your hands too much.

- It can be helpful to use gloves while handling allergens or irritants and to stay away from recognized triggers.

 3. **Hair Care Schedule**:

- Regularly moisturizing the skin with ointments or emollients can help preserve the skin's protective layer and stop moisture loss.

- You can lessen skin irritation by using gentle, fragrance-free cleansers and by not using hot water when taking a bath or shower.

4. **Stress Reduction**:

- Stress-relieving pursuits like physical activity, meditation, or hobbies can enhance general well-being and avert flare-ups of eczema brought on by stress.

5. **Advise and Supervision**:

- Consulting a dermatologist or other healthcare professional regularly can help track eczema symptoms and modify treatment regimens as necessary.

Maintaining a journal to record triggers and flare-ups might offer important information for successfully managing the illness.

Dyshidrotic Eczema sufferers can greatly lessen the frequency and intensity of flare-ups, improving their quality of life and skin health, by being aware of these triggers and taking preventative steps and lifestyle changes in response.

CHAPTER 4

MEDICAL INTERVENTIONS AND TREATMENTS

External corticosteroids:

Topical corticosteroids are frequently used to treat dyshidrotic eczema-related irritation and itching. They function by lowering immunological response, decreasing inflammation, and easing symptoms including itching, swelling, and redness. The strength and formulation of these medications vary based on the severity of the ailment; they might be mild to strong. To prevent possible adverse effects including skin darkening or thinning, you must adhere to your healthcare provider's advice about the frequency and duration of treatment.

Inhibitors of Calcineurin:

An additional family of drugs used to treat dyshidrotic eczema is called calcineurin inhibitors. They function by preventing the immunological reaction that causes skin irritation and inflammation. In contrast to corticosteroids, calcineurin inhibitors are frequently applied to delicate regions such as the face and neck. Some common examples of calcineurin inhibitors are tacrolimus and pimecrolimus. Based on your unique needs, your doctor will decide on the right strength and application schedule.

Antihistamines:

Antihistamines are drugs that lessen allergic reactions and ease itching. They might not be able to cure dyshidrotic eczema directly, but they can help lessen the discomfort brought on by itching. While sedating antihistamines may be advised for use at night, non-drowsy antihistamines are frequently recommended for use during the day. Before beginning any new medicine, always get advice from your healthcare professional, particularly if you have any other medical concerns or are already taking medication.

Emollients and moisturizers:

Managing dyshidrotic eczema requires maintaining moisturized skin. Emollients and moisturizers aid in repairing the skin's protective layer, lessening dryness, and averting additional aggravation. Seek for items that are suitable for sensitive skin, hypoallergenic, and fragrance-free. Regularly moisturize your skin to seal in moisture and shield it from outside aggressors. This is especially important after taking a bath.

Light therapy, or phototherapy:

Phototherapy is the application of regulated UV light dosages to the afflicted skin. For some people with dyshidrotic eczema, this medication can help lessen inflammation, itching, and the frequency of flare-ups. The procedure is usually carried out under medical supervision, and the length and intensity of light exposure will be customized to meet your requirements. For best effects, phototherapy can be used either on its own or in conjunction with other therapies.

Systemic Interventions:

Systemic therapies may be considered when phototherapy and topical medicines are not sufficient. These consist of immunosuppressants, oral corticosteroids, and other drugs that work on the underlying immune response. Because of the possible risks and side effects, these treatments are often only used for severe or refractory cases of dyshidrotic eczema and need to be well-monitored by a healthcare professional.

Biological Treatments:

A more recent class of drugs known as biologic treatments target certain immune system components linked to inflammatory diseases such as dyshidrotic eczema. These drugs are frequently saved for people with severe symptoms or those who have not reacted well to previous therapies. To ensure safety and efficacy, biological medicines must be regularly monitored. They are provided by injection or infusion.

Approaches in Alternative Medicine:

Some people may look into complementary and alternative medicine techniques for treating dyshidrotic eczema, such as acupuncture, herbal therapies, or dietary supplements. Even though these methods might help some people with their symptoms, it's important to talk to your healthcare practitioner about them before implementing them into your treatment plan. Not every alternative therapy has scientific backing, and some can make symptoms worse or interfere with prescription drugs.

Combining Therapies to Get Better Outcomes:

Several therapy modalities combined may be required for the best possible management of dyshidrotic eczema. To address your unique symptoms and causes, your healthcare provider may suggest a combination of systemic treatments, phototherapy, topical drugs, and lifestyle changes. You must adhere to your treatment plan and let your healthcare provider know about any concerns or modifications to your condition.

Handling Hazards and Side Effects:

Every medical therapy and treatment has hazards and adverse consequences. To reduce these, it's important to be aware of them and to collaborate closely with your healthcare provider. Effective side effect management may require routine monitoring, dose adjustments, and lifestyle changes. Make sure to notify your healthcare team as soon as you notice any new or worsening symptoms so they may be appropriately evaluated and managed.

Through a collaborative effort with your healthcare provider, you can create a customized and all-encompassing approach to controlling your dyshidrotic eczema that caters to your specific requirements and concerns.

CHAPTER 5

STRATEGIES FOR SKINCARE AND MANAGEMENT

Careful Skincare Techniques:

- Use gentle cleansers and soaps without fragrances to prevent skin irritation.

- Pat dry your skin softly rather than rubbing it dry with force.

Steer clear of hot water since it can worsen eczema and deplete the skin of its natural oils.

Moisturing and Bathing Methods:

Take quick, warm showers or baths to avoid drying out your skin.

- To seal in moisture, apply moisturizer right away after taking a bath.

- For the best hydration, look for moisturizers that contain ceramides, glycerin, or hyaluronic acid.

Selecting Appropriate Skincare Items:

- Pay attention to labels that say "fragrance-free," "hypoallergenic," and "for sensitive skin."

- Before using new items all over, patch-test them on a tiny section of your body.

Steer clear of products that have harsh chemicals, alcohol, or retinoids as they might irritate skin prone to eczema.

Selected Clothes and Fabrics:

- To lessen irritation, choose breathable, soft materials like silk or cotton.

- Before wearing new clothing, wash it to get rid of any possible allergens.

Steer clear of clothing that is too tight as this may cause friction and skin rashes.

Sun Protection:

- To shield your skin from UV radiation, apply a broad-spectrum sunscreen with an SPF of 30 or above.

- When spending time outside, dress in protective apparel, such as long sleeves and hats.

Seek cover to minimize sun exposure from 10 a.m. to 4 p.m. during the peak sun hours.

Management Strategies for Stress:

- To relieve tension, engage in relaxation exercises like yoga, meditation, or deep breathing.

- Recognise and deal with your life's stressors, such as your job or interpersonal connections.

- For further assistance, think about speaking with a therapist or counselor.

Hygiene of Sleep:

- Create a regular sleep routine and follow it every day, including on the weekends.

Establish a calming evening ritual to assist in de-stressing before bed.

- For the best possible sleep, keep your bedroom quiet, cold, and dark.

Workout and Physical Activity:

- To prevent perspiration, try low-impact activities like yoga, swimming, or strolling.

- After working out, take a shower and moisturize right away to get rid of sweat and avoid dry skin.

- To keep your skin pleasant while working out, dress in breathable, moisture-wicking materials.

Dietary and Nutritional Considerations:

- Continue to eat a well-balanced diet full of nutritious grains, fruits, vegetables, and lean meats.

- Drink lots of water throughout the day to stay hydrated.

- Restrict or stay away from foods like dairy, gluten, and some spices that can cause flare-ups of eczema.

Including Self-Care in Everyday Activities:

- Schedule daily self-care activities that support well-being and relaxation.

Make self-care routines like stress reduction, exercise, a good diet, and skincare a priority.

- To get long-term benefits for your skin and general health, stick to your self-care regimen.

CHAPTER 6

HANDLING EMOTIONAL DIFFICULTIES

Dyshidrotic Eczema's Effect on Mental Health:

Despite being largely a physical ailment, dyshidrotic eczema can have a significant effect on mental health. Feelings of irritation, shame, and even despair or anxiety might result from the constant itching, discomfort, and outward signs. Managing the physical symptoms of the illness constantly can also cause sleep disturbances and increase stress, which exacerbate mental health issues.

Affective Reactions and Coping Mechanisms

People who have dyshidrotic eczema frequently react emotionally in a variety of ways, such as being angry, depressed, frustrated, or low in self-esteem. Creating a regular skincare regimen, avoiding triggers like specific allergies or irritants, practicing relaxation techniques, and asking loved ones or mental health professionals for emotional assistance are a few examples of coping mechanisms. While actively attempting to manage these emotions healthily, it's critical to recognize and validate these feelings.

Resources and Support Systems

Developing a robust support network is essential for the management of dyshidrotic eczema. This can include close friends and family, support networks, and medical professionals who are aware of the illness and can provide both emotional and practical guidance. In addition, there are a plethora of offline and online resources, including forums, instructional materials, and advocacy groups, that can offer insightful information and connections to people going through comparable struggles.

Options for Counselling and Therapy

The emotional toll that dyshidrotic eczema has on a person can be greatly alleviated by counseling and therapy. Psychotherapy, including cognitive-behavioral therapy (CBT), can assist people in recognizing and confronting harmful thought patterns, acquiring coping mechanisms, and enhancing their general emotional health. Seeking guidance from a therapist or counselor with expertise in treating chronic skin problems can offer customized assistance that is suited to the particular difficulties associated with eczema management.

Meditation and Mindfulness Techniques:

Practices like mindfulness and meditation can be very effective in reducing stress and enhancing mental health. Deep breathing, progressive muscle relaxation, and guided visualization are some of the techniques that assist people with dyshidrotic eczema learn to be calm and less anxious. Including these activities in daily life can help people unwind, become more self-aware, and live better overall.

Diarying and Introspection

Processing feelings and monitoring eczema symptoms can be aided by journaling or self-reflection. In addition to offering a sense of release and clarity, writing about thoughts and feelings associated with the illness can help discover patterns or triggers that might make symptoms worse. Frequent self-reflection can help one become more resilient and self-aware by fostering a deeper understanding of their coping strategies and emotional reactions.

Building Hardiness

Developing resilience is crucial to handling the emotional difficulties associated with dyshidrotic eczema. This can entail developing a positive outlook, taking care of oneself, establishing reasonable goals, and asking for help when required. Building flexible coping mechanisms and taking lessons from failures can help people become more resilient and capable of handling the highs and lows of having a chronic skin disease.

Teaching Friends and Family

Informing loved ones and friends about dyshidrotic eczema can help to promote tolerance, compassion, and support. Giving loved ones knowledge about the illness, its signs and symptoms, causes, and available treatments can enable them to provide real support and encouragement. Relationships can be strengthened and a supportive environment can be created for managing eczema-related difficulties through open conversation and experience sharing.

Community Involvement and Advocacy

Being involved in advocacy work and interacting with people who have eczema can be uplifting and empowering. Promoting greater understanding, investigation, and access to care can help those who suffer from dyshidrotic eczema as well as future generations who may have comparable difficulties. Engaging in online communities, events, and support groups can offer inspiration, affirmation, and a sense of community.

Small Victories to Celebrate

Encouraging minor accomplishments, such as having a good skin day, efficiently handling symptoms, or accomplishing a personal goal, is crucial for preserving resilience and drive. No matter how tiny, acknowledging accomplishments promotes positive actions and attitudes, which enhances general well-being and quality of life. It is possible to develop a sense of thankfulness and resilience in the face of adversity by setting aside time to celebrate successes and happy situations.

CHAPTER 7

MODIFICATIONS TO LIFESTYLE FOR THE TREATMENT OF DYSHIDROTIC ECZEMA

Work and Career-Related Issues

There are a few important factors to take into account when managing dyshidrotic eczema at work. First and foremost, it's critical to let your employer know about your condition and explain how it can affect your work as well as any necessary accommodations. For instance, you might need to talk about alternate responsibilities or safety precautions if your employment requires you to wash your hands a lot or exposes you to allergens.

When performing duties that require hand protection, think about using cotton gloves underneath vinyl or latex gloves. To avoid dryness and cracking, keep a moisturizer close at hand and use it frequently. Investigate stress-reduction methods like mindfulness or breathing exercises if stress makes your eczema worse.

Relationships and Social Life

Social interactions and relationships may be impacted by dyshidrotic eczema, particularly if visible symptoms create pain or self-consciousness. You must inform your close friends and family about your condition so that they can provide understanding and support. Select social activities that do not worsen your symptoms; for instance, choose outside activities instead of spending a lot of time in hot, muggy conditions.

Be honest with your loved ones about how your eczema affects your social interactions. Never be afraid to establish limits if particular situations or activities cause flare-ups.

Advice for Travelling

When traveling, one must make special arrangements for dyshidrotic eczema. Stow medicine and moisturizers in travel-sized containers in your carry-on luggage to guarantee access during flights. To reduce irritation, use skincare products that are mild and fragrance-free. When visiting a new region, consider the potential effects of the weather on your skin and modify your skincare regimen accordingly.

If you think you might require medical attention while traveling, look into the local hospitals. Think about getting travel insurance that pays for treatments connected to eczema or other pre-existing diseases.

Handling Exacerbations and Flares

Dyshidrotic eczema flare-ups can be difficult but controllable. Recognize and stay away from triggers, such as allergies, stress, and particular meals. To prevent infection, moisturize your skin thoroughly and refrain from scratching.

For individualized flare-up management techniques, such as prescription medicine or phototherapy, speak with your dermatologist. To monitor flare-ups and spot trends or causes, keep a journal.

Managing Sleep

Getting enough sleep is crucial for controlling dyshidrotic eczema. Establish a calming nighttime routine that includes moisturizing and light skincare. Use pajamas and bedding that are hypoallergenic to reduce inflammation.

Use topical remedies or antihistamines before bed if itchy skin keeps you awake.

Maintaining a regular sleep schedule and setting up a peaceful, distraction-free sleeping environment are two ways to practice excellent sleep hygiene.

Monetary Factors

Financial issues for managing dyshidrotic eczema may include prescription drug costs, dermatologist visits, and skincare product purchases. To cut costs, look into insurance coverage options and generic pharmaceutical alternatives.

Seek out patient aid programs provided by non-profits or pharmaceutical firms, as these may offer funding for eczema treatments. Make skincare purchases a regular component of your budget, giving top priority to items that your dermatologist has suggested.

Handling Misunderstandings and Stigma

People who have dyshidrotic eczema may experience stigma or misinterpretations from others. Gain knowledge about the illness so that you can confidently respond to inquiries and disbeliefs. Be in the company of people who are understanding and appreciative of your experiences.

Join online forums or eczema advocacy groups to meet people going through similar things and exchange experiences. Recall that your skin condition does not determine your value.

Interacting with Medical Professionals

Having good contact with medical professionals is essential to controlling dyshidrotic eczema. Maintain a log of your symptoms, triggers, and responses to treatment so that you are ready for appointments. Inquire about possible side effects, treatment alternatives, and your condition.

Get in quick contact with your dermatologist to discuss any worries or modifications to your situation. Adhere to your treatment plan religiously and make follow-up appointments on time.

Including Eczema Management in Everyday Activities

Making self-care a priority, avoiding irritants, and developing regular skincare routines are all essential to managing eczema in daily life. Ensure that skincare supplies are easily accessible whether traveling, at work, or home.

To reduce flare-ups, use stress-reduction methods like yoga or meditation.

Include mild activity in your regimen to enhance general health and lessen stress, which can aggravate eczema symptoms. When necessary, ask family members and medical experts for assistance.

Establishing Reasonable Expectations and Goals

Having realistic objectives and goals is essential to properly managing dyshidrotic eczema. Recognize that treating eczema is a lifelong process that may require trying out various remedies. Concentrate on attainable objectives like lessening flare-ups or enhancing skin moisture.

Acknowledge minor accomplishments on your path to managing eczema and ask for help when things get tough. Your healthcare team can help you make any necessary adjustments to your treatment plans and goals.

CHAPTER 8
PARTICULAR ATTENTION TO VARIOUS AGE GROUPS
Children's Dyshidrotic Eczema

Children's and adults' experiences with dyshidrotic eczema are frequently dissimilar. It is essential to use gentle skincare products because the skin is more sensitive and prone to discomfort. Moisturizers and emollients are essential for controlling symptoms and averting flare-ups. It's also critical to recognize and stay away from triggers, which can include particular foods, materials, or surroundings. A pediatric dermatologist can be consulted regularly to ensure appropriate care and therapy modifications as the child develops.

Adolescents and Teens

Teens and adolescents may experience particular difficulties with dyshidrotic eczema because of changes in hormones, elevated stress, and social pressures. It's critical to promote honest dialogue regarding their situation and offer emotional support. Symptoms can be effectively managed by highlighting the significance of regular skincare regimens, stress-reduction strategies, and healthy lifestyle choices.

Working professionals and adults

It can be difficult for adults with dyshidrotic eczema to strike a balance between their professional and personal obligations, particularly in stressful job settings. Time management tactics, regular exercise, and mindfulness are examples of stress management practices that can be helpful. In addition to using hypoallergenic skincare products, encouraging a positive work atmosphere, and taking pauses to apply moisturizers can all help with symptoms and general well-being.

Senior People

Older people may have more health issues and less elastic skin, which increases their risk of developing skin infections and dyshidrotic eczema problems. It's important to practice gentle skincare, enough hydration, and regular skin examinations. Results and quality of life can be enhanced by addressing mobility or cognitive issues and making necessary adjustments to treatment regimens.

Handling Eczema and Pregnancy

The symptoms of dyshidrotic eczema might change throughout pregnancy; some women may observe improvements, while others may experience flare-ups. To guarantee the mother's and the child's safety, it is crucial to speak with a healthcare professional before beginning or modifying any treatments. It is crucial to emphasize gentle skincare, stress-reduction methods, and keeping an eye out for any allergic responses or changes in symptoms during pregnancy.

Guidance for Parents of Children with Eczema

To effectively treat their child's dyshidrotic eczema, parents are essential. Establishing a calming nighttime regimen, utilizing fragrance-free and hypoallergenic products, and educating kids about good skincare from an early age can all have a big impact. Establishing a supportive atmosphere can also be facilitated by educating teachers, carers, and other adults engaged in the child's life about eczema triggers and management.

Difficulties in Education and Schools

Dyshidrotic eczema in children and teenagers can cause discomfort, irritation, and possibly even low self-esteem, which can make school difficult. Establishing a supportive and inclusive school environment can be achieved through closely collaborating with school personnel to implement a care plan, giving classmates education on eczema, and granting access to moisturizers and medications as needed.

Eczema and Career Development

Proactive self-care techniques are necessary to manage dyshidrotic eczema while pursuing career objectives. Succeeding in the workplace can be attributed to putting stress management first, keeping a good work-life balance, and asking for concessions when needed. Being open and honest about eczema and its effects with coworkers or bosses might help to build understanding and support.

Managing Eczema with Grace

Managing dyshidrotic eczema may need to be adjusted as people age to account for changes in skin health and general well-being. It's crucial to hydrate, modify skincare regimens to fit aging skin, and do regular skin examinations. Encouraging healthy aging with eczema can be facilitated by seeking advice from healthcare experts regarding medication management and lifestyle adjustments.

Eczema and Family Planning

It's crucial for people with dyshidrotic eczema who want to start a family to speak with medical professionals. Important factors to take into account include ensuring that drugs are safe to take while pregnant or nursing, controlling stress, and sticking to a regular skincare regimen. Managing family planning while having eczema can be facilitated by the assistance of partners, family members, and medical specialists.

When managing dyshidrotic eczema, every age group has unique considerations and obstacles. Through comprehension of these distinct requirements and execution of customized tactics, people can proficiently handle their illness and enhance their standard of living during various phases of life.

CHAPTER 9

INVESTIGATIONS AND ADVANCEMENTS IN ECZEMA THERAPY

Recent Research Findings:

Keep yourself informed on the most recent discoveries in the field of dyshidrotic eczema research. This entails being aware of the root causes, stressors, and prospective therapeutic advances. New routes, like immune system regulation, skin barrier repair, and the impact of environmental variables in worsening symptoms, are being regularly explored by researchers.

Treatment techniques:

Treatment techniques for dyshidrotic eczema have undergone encouraging developments. These consist of phototherapy, calcineurin inhibitors, and topical corticosteroids. Biologic treatments that target particular immune responses are another example of recent developments. For improved symptom management, combination treatments and lifestyle adjustments are being investigated.

New Therapies and Technologies

JAK inhibitors and monoclonal antibodies are two examples of new treatments that could be useful in treating severe cases of dyshidrotic eczema. Keep a watch on these treatments. Furthermore, cutting-edge methods for remotely monitoring and managing symptoms are made possible by technology like wearable sensors and telemedicine platforms, which improve patient convenience and care.

The significance of clinical trials in assessing the safety and effectiveness of novel treatments for dyshidrotic eczema cannot be overstated. By taking part in these trials, patients can have access to state-of-the-art treatments and further medical understanding of the treatment of eczema.

Genomic Research and Personalised Medicine:

Research on genomes reveals potential hereditary susceptibilities to dyshidrotic eczema. Personalized medicine techniques are made possible by this knowledge, which allows for improved outcomes by customizing medicines based on a patient's genetic composition and unique illness characteristics.

Patient-Driven Research Initiatives:

Take part in research projects that allow people who have dyshidrotic eczema to share their knowledge and perspectives. Collaboration between patients, medical professionals, and researchers is encouraged by these programs, which promote patient-centered care and enhance treatment results.

The Role of Artificial Intelligence in Eczema Care:

From aiding in diagnosis through image recognition algorithms to forecasting the course of the disease and the effectiveness of treatment, artificial intelligence (AI) is becoming more and more involved in the management of eczema. Healthcare professionals can make better decisions and tailor treatment regimens for patients with dyshidrotic eczema with the use of AI-driven technologies.

Global Initiatives to Raise Awareness of Eczema

These initiatives seek to lower the stigma associated with eczema, raise public knowledge of the condition, and facilitate access to efficient treatments. Global eczema management policies and resources are advocated for, and patient support networks are strengthened, through events like World Eczema Day and educational campaigns.

Prospects for the Future of Eczema Management:

With continued research, technology improvements, and cooperative efforts throughout the scientific community, the future of eczema management is bright. Personalized treatment algorithms, precision medicine, and targeted therapeutics have the potential to improve outcomes and quality of life for people with dyshidrotic eczema.

Collaboration in Scientific Communities:

Promoting innovation in eczema management, exchanging best practices, and expanding knowledge all depend on collaboration within scientific communities.

Dermatologists, immunologists, geneticists, and patient advocates work together in multidisciplinary teams to provide holistic care and advance our understanding of and ability to treat dyshidrotic eczema in its entirety.

CHAPTER 10
GAINING SELF- AND OTHER-EMPOWERMENT

Education as an Empowerment Tool

When it comes to empowering people with dyshidrotic eczema, education is essential. It is essential to comprehend the illness, its causes, symptoms, and potential therapies. With this information, people may successfully interact with healthcare practitioners, make educated decisions about their health, and actively engage in their treatment plans.

Promoting Awareness of Eczema

The goal of advocacy work is to increase public knowledge about dyshidrotic eczema. This entails raising awareness of the difficulties experienced by eczema sufferers among the general public, legislators, and medical professionals. It also entails encouraging research into potential cures and fighting for more accessible healthcare and reasonably priced prescription drugs.

Establishing Networks of Support

Support groups offer people with dyshidrotic eczema a sense of community, comprehension, and encouragement. These networks might consist of loved ones, close friends, support groups, internet forums, and medical professionals that give helpful advice on managing the disease as well as emotional support and experience sharing.

Compassion and Empathy in the Medical Field

When treating patients with dyshidrotic eczema in a medical context, empathy and compassion are crucial. Healthcare professionals should pay close attention to patients, verify their experiences, address any concerns they may have, and work together to create individualized treatment programs. Empathy increases patient outcomes, builds trust, and raises the standard of care in general.

The Path of Personal Growth

Dyshidrotic eczema sufferers frequently embark on a personal development path. This path may involve embracing a positive outlook, practicing self-care practices, building resilience, learning how to manage both physical and emotional difficulties, and creating reasonable goals. Every step of this path advances personal development and empowerment.

Motivational Tales of Eczema Fighters

Telling encouraging tales of people who have effectively controlled their dyshidrotic eczema can give hope, inspiration, and support to those who are going through comparable difficulties. These tales encourage people to continue taking the initiative in controlling their conditions and achieving their objectives because they demonstrate resiliency, tenacity, and the possibility of favorable results.

Honouring a Variety of Experiences

People with dyshidrotic eczema come in many ages, backgrounds, and lifestyles. Honoring these varied experiences fosters inclusivity, understanding, and empathy. It also fosters teamwork in the search for creative solutions and supportive tactics that address the particular requirements of every person.

Being Responsible for Your Health

Proactive self-management techniques, like keeping a skincare regimen, recognizing and avoiding triggers, leading a healthy lifestyle, following recommended treatments, going to routine checkups, and being honest with medical professionals, are all part of taking responsibility for one's health. People who feel empowered actively manage their health and make decisions that are best for their overall well-being.

Propaganda Hope and Positivity

Keeping an optimistic attitude and fostering optimism can make a significant difference for those with dyshidrotic eczema. Resilience, stress reduction, and general well-being are all enhanced by positivity. For all those impacted by the illness, a more upbeat and uplifting atmosphere can be created by sharing success stories, fostering self-care routines, and building a strong community.

Building a Future Free of Stigma Around Eczema

To eradicate the stigma attached to dyshidrotic eczema, people, communities, medical professionals, and legislators must work together. This entails raising awareness, dispelling myths, fighting for fairness in opportunities and treatment, and cultivating a climate of tolerance, compassion, and support for those who suffer from eczema. To eradicate stigma in the future, there must be constant learning, honest communication, and inclusive behaviors across all spheres of society.

We can empower people with dyshidrotic eczema, foster empathy and understanding, and work towards a future where everyone may thrive regardless of their health condition by addressing these important areas.

www.ingramcontent.com/pod-product-compliance
Lightning Source LLC
Chambersburg PA
CBHW061254250726
48653CB00002B/655